HOLISTIC HEALTH REVOLUTION

Reach Ideal Weight, Enjoy a Balanced Diet, Improve Sleep, and Gain Transformative Overall Vitality

By

RABI NARAYAN MOHANTY

Dedication

This book is dedicated to my beloved Late father, Mohan Charan Mohanty

Your unwavering support, inspiration, and example of discipline and health have been the guiding light in my journey from illness to wellness. Your memory and teachings continue to inspire me every day. Thank you for being my mentor, my role model, and my greatest supporter. This work is a tribute to your enduring legacy and the profound impact you've had on my life.

YOUR FREE GIFT

Scan the QR code below to receive your FREE GIFT!

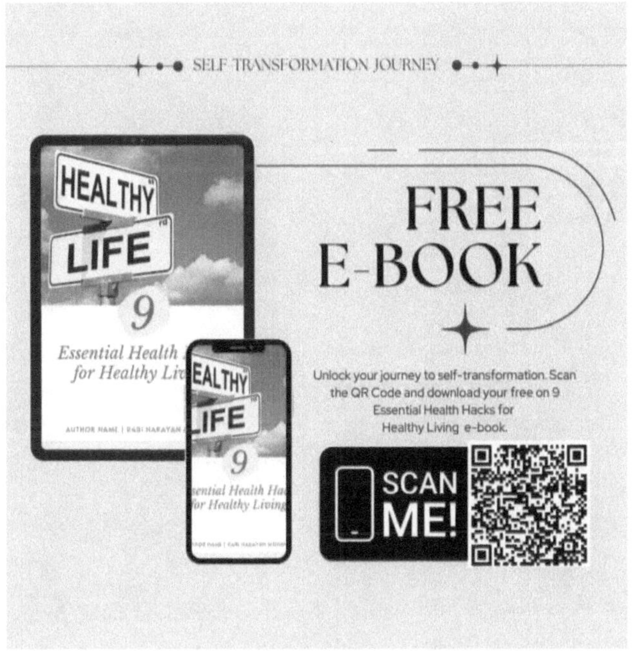

Why Is This Book For You?

After going through this life-changing transformation, I now understand the pain and challenges of living with chronic health issues. My mission is to help others avoid the suffering I endured and embrace a healthier life through small but consistent lifestyle changes. Prevention is always better than cure.

This book is more than just a guide to weight loss or balanced nutrition—it is the roadmap I followed to achieve wellness.

If you are seeking a holistic approach to your health, with a focus on adopting healthy habits and making better choices, then this book is for you.

It offers a proven method for achieving your wellness goals, just as I did. With the right mindset and determination, you can change your life, and I am here to guide you along the way.

TABLE OF CONTENTS

Chapter 1

My Journey from Illness to Wellness

This book is not just a collection of health tips; it is my personal story of transformation, filled with struggle, pain, inspiration, and, ultimately, triumph. My journey from illness to wellness began in my childhood when I was carefree and enjoyed life to the fullest. I never worried about chronic illnesses or health issues. However, everything changed when, at the age of 12, I was diagnosed with acute sinusitis, marked by a polyp in my nostril. This led to frequent respiratory blockages, severe colds, sneezing, and sometimes high fevers. Even the smallest change in weather or exposure to dust triggered these episodes, along with intense headaches.

Despite being advised by a specialist to exercise and manage my condition, I did not make the necessary lifestyle changes at that time. As a result, I suffered from sinusitis and its associated complications for over two decades—a crucial period of my life.

During my academic years and early professional life, I developed gastrointestinal disorders, including IBS, severe gastric issues, and piles. Stress, an unhealthy lifestyle, lack of exercise, and poor dietary habits compounded my health problems. Frequent doctor visits and the constant use of antibiotics and painkillers provided temporary relief but led to new health challenges.

The medications themselves contributed to my worsening condition, especially gastrointestinal issues, and I found myself trapped in a cycle of illness, frustration, and isolation.

But life has a way of guiding us toward change. My turning point came when I was exposed to concepts like healthy habits, lifestyle changes, and balanced nutrition. Most importantly, I was inspired by my father, a true role model in fitness and disciplined living. My father maintained a healthy lifestyle throughout his life, dedicating 120 minutes a day to rigorous exercise, including morning and evening walks totaling around 6 km.

His consistent schedule, nutritious eating, and avoidance of processed foods helped him stay fit and free from chronic diseases.

After years of prompting from him, I finally took the first step toward my own transformation. I began waking up early, drinking lukewarm water in the morning, and committing to 45 minutes of exercise, including pranayama (breathing exercises). Gradually, I improved my dietary choices, hydration habits, and overall lifestyle.

With the inspiration of my father and the guidance of a wellness coach, I successfully lost 17 pounds of excess fat and achieved my ideal weight. More importantly, I freed myself from the health challenges that had plagued me for years.

This transformation was not easy—it was painful, emotional, and challenging. But it was worth every moment. I share this story not just to inspire but to connect with those who are struggling with their own health challenges. I know what it's like to suffer, but I also know that recovery is possible.

When I began writing this book, my beloved father had already passed away, tragically lost in a road accident during his regular morning walk. His unwavering discipline, honesty, and integrity continue to inspire me every day.

He lived a life of fitness and health, never requiring hospitalization and remaining active until his last day. His memory motivates me to share my story with the world.

Chapter 2

Mastering Ideal Weight

"You didn't gain all your weight in one day; you won't lose it in one day. Be patient with yourself."

- Jenna Wolfe

➢ **Understanding the Significance of Achieving an Ideal Weight:**

"Have you ever wondered why the concept of 'ideal weight' is so central to discussions about health? What if achieving this balance could significantly transform not only your physical health but also your quality of life?"

Do you know the worldwide obesity rate has nearly doubled since 1980?

Achieving and maintaining an ideal weight is an important component of overall wellness. Achieving and maintaining an ideal weight is more than just a number on the scale—it's a vital factor in enhancing overall health and wellness. Understanding the significance of this balance can provide profound insights into how our body functions and how we can optimize our health for a better quality of life.

Maintaining an ideal weight can help reduce the risk of various chronic degenerative diseases such as diabetes, heart disease, hypertension, arthritis, Parkinson's disease and etc.

Real-Life Transformation: A Saint's Journey to Health

Throughout my journey, I've come across many inspiring stories of individuals who achieved remarkable health transformations after reaching their ideal weight. One such story is about a saint who had dedicated his entire life to spiritual devotion. He was a keynote speaker on a regional television channel, regularly delivering spiritual talks and traveling extensively between various ashrams for prayers and discourses.

However, his busy schedule and sedentary lifestyle began to take a toll on his health. He faced numerous challenges, including obesity, diabetes, and high blood pressure. His body had accumulated a significant amount of fat, particularly around his belly, and his overall shape was irregular due to the fat deposits. To manage his diabetes, he relied on insulin and other medications prescribed by his doctors. Despite this, his health continued to deteriorate, primarily due to his sedentary habits and unhealthy food choices.

During one of his stays at a devotee's house, the saint was introduced to a wellness and lifestyle coach. The coach conducted a comprehensive body scan to assess his health parameters, which revealed alarming results: high body weight, excessive visceral fat, and poor overall health. Realizing the seriousness of his condition, the saint decided to make a change.

Under the guidance of the wellness coach, he adopted a new lifestyle. His diet was completely revamped, focusing on balanced nutrition and appropriate supplements. In addition to this, a tailored exercise plan was implemented. Through consistent effort and disciplined adherence to this new lifestyle, the saint gradually achieved his ideal weight and restored balance to his body's parameters.

Today, he lives a healthy, disease-free life, free from obesity, diabetes, and high blood pressure. His transformation is a powerful testament to the life-changing effects of achieving one's ideal weight through commitment, proper guidance, and a holistic approach to health.

According to the obesity statistics data published in Forbes Health:

Obesity is linked to 30% to 53% of new diabetes cases in the U.S. every year, per research in the *Journal of the American Heart Association*.

- **Medical costs for people with obesity in the U.S. tend to be 30% to 40% higher than those for people without obesity**

Nowadays, health practitioners are suggesting losing weight and achieving the ideal weight, especially for patients with arthritis, knee or joint pain, diabetes, or cardiovascular disease.

The rise of obesity is a wake-up call. In recent times, a shadow has been cast over our global health landscape. According to the World Obesity Atlas 2022, published by the World Obesity Federation, a comprehensive and reputable source of health data, it predicts that one billion people globally, including 1 in 5 women and 1 in 7 men, will be living with obesity by 2030.

Additionally, the 10th edition of the IDF Diabetes Atlas reports "a continued global increase in type 2 diabetes, for which obesity is a key driver."

The frequency of obesity, and in response to that, the frequency of type 2 diabetes is on a steady upward trend. This is not just a statistic; it's a serious warning bell for the state of our collective well-being.

A 2022 study in Frontiers in Cardiovascular Medicine found people with obesity with higher waist-to-height ratios had a 71% higher risk of cancer than those with lower waist-to-height ratios.

Benefits of Achieving Ideal Weight:-

By achieving and maintaining an ideal weight, you can reduce the risk of various chronic degenerative diseases like type 2 diabetes, some types of cancer, heart disease, arthritis, Parkinson's disease, etc. An ideal weight contributes to healthier blood pressure and overall heart health.

Carrying less excess weight results in less strain on the joints and muscles of the body, helping with free movement and performing activities. As a result, it can reduce joint-related issues and improve joint health.

Achieving an ideal weight can also help improve gut health, which boosts the immunity of the body.

Achieving an ideal weight not only helps to enhance your physical health but also enhances your mental and behavioral health. It can boost self-confidence and self-esteem. It can help manage stress levels, leading to improved mental well-being.

It can improve sleep quality and increase the energy level of the body, leading to a more active and fulfilling life. I have already explained in my story that after reaching an ideal weight and maintaining a healthy, active lifestyle, I was able to maintain amazing gut health, including overall holistic health.

Research says that nowadays, in every field, priority is given to achieving an ideal weight before proceeding further. For example, health practitioners are advising their patients to lose excess weight as a part of their treatment, especially for patients with knee and joint pain, cardiovascular disease, diabetes, etc. The same priority is given in sports, the entertainment field, aviation, defense, and most highly responsible sectors.

"I have come across so many people who experience chronic joint pain and knee pain. Their health experts

advised all of them to lose excess body weight as a top priority."

So, the benefits of achieving an ideal weight are far more than physical health. They cover mental, emotional, and social well-being, making it a crucial aspect of holistic wellness.

However, maintaining a Healthy weight can be a challenging task with the abundance of high-caloric, low-nutrient-dense foods and the sedentary lifestyle of the human race including the availability of misinformation related to it.

So, the benefits of achieving an ideal weight go far beyond physical health. They encompass mental, emotional, and social well-being, making it a crucial aspect of holistic wellness.

➢ **Practical Tips on How to Achieve the Ideal Weight and Maintain a Healthy & Active Life:**

1. **Finding Ideal Weight & Setting a Healthy Goal:**

The first step of the journey is to find the ideal weight of the body. By using a standard weighing machine or body composition monitor, we can find the weight of the body, and then, using a measuring tape, find out the height in inch.

Ideal body weight was initially introduced by Ben J. Devine in 1974 to allow estimation of drug clearance in obese patients; researchers have since shown that the metabolism of certain drugs relates more to ideal body weight than total body weight.

The Devine formula for calculating ideal body weight in adults is as follows:

Male ideal body weight = 110 lb + 2.0 lb × (height (cm) – 152).

Female ideal body weight = 100 lb + 2.0 lb × (height (cm) – 152).

Or, we can also find out the ideal weight by a simple rule of thumb as follows:

Ideal weight in pounds = 5 x BMI + (BMI divided by 5) x (Height in inches minus 60)

Now, the difference between the actual weight measured on the weighing machine and the ideal weight calculated from any of the above formulas will be the weight to lose or gain.

That means if the actual weight is more than the calculated ideal weight, then it needs weight loss, and if the actual weight is less than the calculated ideal weight, then it needs weight gain.

The main things contributing to our body weight are fat, muscle mass, bone, and water. So, a healthy weight loss process means losing unwanted fat, not muscle mass. Losing muscle mass is not a healthy sign during a weight loss journey.

To know the body parameters like Fat %, Muscle %, Bone Density, Water % for better analyzing the weight loss journey, you can use any Body Scanner Machine.

After finding the ideal body weight, we have to set our goal of how much weight (i.e., unwanted fat) to lose by adopting a healthy weight loss process. Our goal for achieving ideal weight should be specific, measurable, time-bound, and realistic.

For example, after finding the ideal weight, find out how much weight is to lose with reference to the actual body weight measured. Then, fix a time period, i.e., in how many months the said weight has to lose. Then, accordingly, a daily action plan should be made related to a healthy and balanced eating plan, a daily schedule for following a healthy lifestyle, a daily exercise schedule, etc.

Slow weight loss is often more sustainable and beneficial because it allows your body to adapt to gradual and lasting changes to a healthy lifestyle and eating habits. This can lead to long-term weight maintenance. By a slow weight loss process, there will be no loss of muscle, which is a healthy sign for body metabolism and overall health.

The rate of weight loss depends on the genetic, physiological & psychological pattern of the body. So, how much weight will have to lose in a month vary from individual to individual. Remember that everyone's weight loss journey is unique, and what works for one person may not work for another.

It's essential to find an approach that fits your individual needs and preferences. The weight loss process is a challenging journey; it requires patience, determination, and a strong mindset. But to achieve great wellness results, it is a small challenge. Focus on making healthy, long-term changes to your diet and exercise routine rather than resorting to extreme measures.

It is better to consult with a healthcare professional or registered dietitian to create a personalized weight loss plan tailored to your needs and goals.

The golden rule for achieving an ideal weight is the 80-20 rule. That means 80% nutrition and 20% exercise, along with a 100% mindset, are the fundamental principles for achieving a healthy weight.

2.Making a Healthy and Balanced Eating Plan to Achieve Ideal Weight:–

One of the most vital steps in achieving a Ideal weight is to make a Healthy eating plan. A Healthy & Balanced diet is a prime requisite for weight loss.

In our healthy eating plan, we should incorporate a variety of nutrient-dense and low-calorie foods such as fruits, green vegetables, whole grains, lean protein, and healthy fats. The main goal of our balanced eating plan, which has a high nutritious and low-calorie diet, is to keep ourselves feeling full & satisfied, along with preventing overeating & weight gain. Our diet should be a mix of protein, healthy carbs, fats, vitamins, minerals, & fiber.

To reach the target of a healthy weight, we should adopt a 5-meal plan instead of 3. Generally, we adopt breakfast, lunch, and dinner as our 3-meal plan. But we usually get hungry about every 3 to 4 hours. So, instead of a 3-meal plan, we can add 2 healthy snacks: one between breakfast & lunch (i.e., at 10 to 11 A.M.) & another between lunch & dinner (i.e., at 4 to 5 P.M.). In these 2 snacks, we can have anything from fruits, salads, eggs, dry fruits, sprouts, etc.

More focus should be on our breakfast. Generally, people are skipping their breakfast during their weight loss process, which is the wrong approach. Skipping breakfast is not a healthy weight loss process. After fasting for around 10 to 12 hours, we eat breakfast (it is for breaking our fast). If we skip breakfast, we may eat more due to hunger, which results in weight gain.

As per global nutrition philosophy, every meal, including breakfast, should have balanced nutrition (it should consist of 30% protein, 40% carbohydrates, & 30% healthy fats along with fiber, vitamins, & minerals). Half of our plate should have fruits & vegetables, 1/4 of the plate should have lean protein, and the remaining 1/4 should have carbohydrates.

Accordingly, we should plan our 5 meals in advance to help ourselves avoid frequent & unhealthy eating.

Another vital part of the eating plan is staying hydrated throughout the day by drinking adequate water relative to body weight, which will help with digestion and make it easier to lose weight.

3. Adequate Regular Exercise:

As we have already discussed above, our diet plan should be more nutritious and less caloric to achieve the target of 80% nutrition on a regular basis. Similarly, to achieve the target of 20% exercise, we need to make a habit of doing at least 30 minutes of regular moderate-intensity exercise, such as brisk walking, jogging, cycling, yoga, Zumba dance, etc. By exercising on most days of the week, we can burn calories, boost our metabolism, and build muscle mass, which helps keep us fit & healthy. This habit can help us lose weight efficiently.

4. Get Enough Sound Sleep:

A sound sleep of 7-8 hours daily is a healthy habit to help regulate our metabolism and appetite. Quality sleep of 7-8 hours plays a vital role in weight loss and overall health. For this, our dinner should be at least 2 hours before sleep. No water should be taken at least 1 hour before sleep.

5. Adopting a Healthy Lifestyle:-

As per the WHO, a "healthy lifestyle is a way of living that lowers the risk of being seriously ill or dying early". By adopting a healthy lifestyle, we can not only lose excess weight but also prevent various lifestyle diseases like coronary heart disease, cancer and diabetes, etc.

A healthy lifestyle comprises adopting the habits of making the right food choices (i.e., taking less caloric and nutritious food and avoiding high-calorie junk foods), drinking adequate water daily at the right time with the right posture, getting adequate quality sleep with an early-to-bed and early-to-rise schedule, adopting a balanced nutritional diet, exercising daily, adopting a positive mindset and thoughts for lowering stress, and associating with like-minded positive people, etc.

➤ **Conclusion: Achieving Your Ideal Weight**

It is well understood that achieving an ideal body weight is a key prerequisite for healthy living. Rising obesity rates have become a global wake-up call, underscoring the urgent need for individuals to take control of their health. By reaching your ideal weight, you significantly reduce the risk of chronic metabolic diseases, improving both longevity and quality of life.

However, achieving and maintaining your ideal weight is far more than just hitting a number on the scale—it's about enhancing your overall wellness. This journey, though challenging, begins with a positive, focused mindset and a commitment to long-term health. The principles outlined in this chapter guide you towards that goal, but success hinges on approaching them with discipline and consistency.

Remember, the path to your ideal weight isn't just about shedding pounds—it's about cultivating habits that will serve you for a lifetime. Stay patient, stay focused, and embrace this process as an investment in your healthiest self.

As you continue this journey, stay committed to consistency and celebrates every small victory along the way. This chapter has provided the tools and insights you need to get started, but always listen to your body and adjust as necessary.

Let's now explore the next chapter to uncover the profound impact of a balanced diet, which will not only support your weight goals but also enhance your overall well-being.

Key Takeaways:-

❖ It is understood that achieving an ideal weight is the prime requisite for holistic wellness. Research says that obesity is the key driver of increasing type 2 diabetes and other chronic degenerative diseases.

❖ By achieving and maintaining an ideal weight, you can reduce the risk of various chronic degenerative diseases like type 2 diabetes, some types of cancer, heart disease, arthritis, Parkinson's disease, etc.

❖ To achieve an ideal weight, it is necessary to follow some practical tips with a 100% positive mindset, patience and consistency.

❖ After finding the ideal body weight using the Devine formula, we have to set our goal of how much weight (i.e., unwanted fat) to lose by adopting a healthy weight loss process. Our goal for achieving an ideal weight should be Specific, Measurable, Time-Bound, and Realistic.

❖ After setting the ideal weight goal, the next step is to make a healthy eating plan with a variety of nutrient-dense and low-calorie foods.

❖ Half of each eating plate should consist of a variety of fruits and vegetables, 1/4 of the plate should have lean protein, and the remaining 1/4 should have complex carbohydrates.

❖ Hydrating ourselves throughout the day by drinking adequate water relative to body weight will help with better digestion and make it easier to lose weight.

❖ An ideal weight journey requires 80% nutrition and 20% exercise to achieve holistic wellness.

❖ We have to make a habit of doing at least 30 minutes of regular moderate-intensity exercise such as brisk walking, jogging, cycling, yoga, Zumba dance, etc., to burn calories, boost our metabolism, build muscle mass, lose weight easily, and make ourselves fit and healthy.

❖ A sound sleep of 7-8 hours daily is a healthy habit to help achieve an ideal weight by regulating our metabolism and appetite.

❖ Adopting a healthy lifestyle comprises healthy food choices, daily exercise, maintaining the right time to eat meals, getting adequate quality sleep with an early-to-bed and early-to-rise routine, adopting a positive mindset and thoughts to lower stress, and associating with like-minded positive people to make your ideal weight journey easier.

❖ The weight loss process is a challenging journey; it requires patience, determination and strong mindset.

❖ It is better to consult with a healthcare professional or registered dietitian to create a personalized weight loss plan tailored to your needs and goals.

CHAPTER 3

THE POWER OF BALANCED DIET

"The food you eat can be either the safest and most powerful form of medicine or the slowest form of poison."

- Ann Wigmore

➢ Introduction:

Generally, when we feel hungry, we eat food. But we do not focus on our food choices, whether they are healthy or not. The food we are eating is not intended to just fulfill our hunger; rather, it should ensure that we get all the nutrients required for our body on a daily basis to remain healthy and active. In earlier times, our elders lived long, healthy lives with the help of natural, unprocessed foods only. We have heard an important fact that "food is medicine." But due to the abnormal rise in population, changing environment, degradation in the quality of food production, and the rising demand for junk foods in the market, this has led to an unhealthy life.

A balanced diet is not just about eating a variety of foods; it's about understanding how to nourish ourselves in a way that supports our physical health while also enhancing our mental and emotional states. Just as our daily work determines our future results, similarly, the diet we consume daily determines our future health. Basically, a balanced diet is a combination of various nutrients in proper proportions, as required by our body's calorie intake. In this chapter, we will focus on the concept of a balanced diet, what essential nutrients are and their functions for holistic wellness, how to design our balanced plate of meals considering the concept of a balanced diet, the various benefits of a balanced diet, and the importance of mindful eating for holistic wellness.

> **Concept of a Balanced Diet:**

The basic concept of a balanced diet is to consume nutrient-dense and less caloric foods. Our daily food should be a balanced diet, which means it should consist of macronutrients, micronutrients, and phytonutrients. Macronutrients are one of the key nutrients in our daily balanced diet. Proteins, carbohydrates, and fats are called macronutrients. Vitamins and minerals are micronutrients. Fiber and antioxidants are phytonutrients.

As per the concept of global nutrition philosophy, our body needs a daily balanced diet consisting of 40% carbohydrates, 30% healthy fats, 30% protein, and 25 grams of fiber. A balanced diet is somewhat personalized, so these percentages of macronutrients in the diet can vary slightly depending on age, sex, body weight, individual needs, goals, and health conditions. For example, athletes may require more protein, while those with specific dietary restrictions or weight loss programs might adjust fat or carbohydrate intake accordingly.

The primary intention is to ensure that every meal contributes to our overall health and wellness by providing essential nutrients with fewer calories. A balanced diet supports the body's metabolic functions, promotes energy, and helps to prevent various chronic diseases.

➢ **Essential Nutrients and Their Functions for Wellness:-**

1. **Proteins:-**

• Protein is the most vital nutrient for our body. It is the building block of our body. Protein is essential for building and repairing tissues, including muscles, and is important for immune function and the production of enzymes and hormones.

• Proteins can be sourced from both plants and animals (i.e., from meat, poultry, fish, eggs, dairy, legumes, beans, whole grains, nuts, and seeds). However, plant protein is highly effective compared to animal protein. Protein provides amino acids that are not produced by our body on its own. We can get all of the amino acids we need from either plants or meat. The main differentiating factor is what else is included in those foods besides the proteins. In general, eating a wide variety of foods, especially whole, unprocessed foods, helps **us** get the healthiest balanced nutrition.

The Recommended Dietary Allowance (RDA) for protein is a modest 0.36 grams per pound of body weight. The RDA is the amount of a nutrient you need to meet your basic nutritional requirements. To determine your daily protein intake, you can multiply your weight in pounds by 0.36.

To determine your daily protein intake:

Multiply your weight in pounds by 0.36 grams.

For example, if you weigh 150 pounds:

150 pounds×0.36 grams/pound=54 grams of protein

2. Carbohydrates:

- Carbohydrates are the body's primary source of energy. They ensure adequate energy for the brain, muscles, and cells. Therefore, it's important to include enough carbohydrates in your diet every day to replace what you've used. It is recommended that you get about 40% of your calories from whole grains, beans, vegetables, and fruits. Avoid carbohydrates from food sources like the sugary, starchy kinds you find in baked goods, soda, and candy. Complex carbohydrates are generally considered healthier than simple carbohydrates because they provide more nutrition. Complex carbohydrates are broken down more slowly, which can help prevent blood sugar spikes. They also contain fiber and bran, which can help with digestion. Brown rice, whole-grain pasta, bread, cereals, apples, oatmeal, beans, lentils, and dried peas are examples of food sources for complex carbs.

3. Fats:-

- Healthy Fats or Dietary Fats help to store energy for the body. Dietary Fats support Heart, Brain & Joint Health, cell functions. Fats are vital for absorbing fat-soluble vitamins (A, D, E, and K).

- Dietary Fats or Healthy Fats shall be saturated, polysaturated & Mono saturated. Too much intake of dietary fats will be bad for body. Source of Dietary fats are Olive Oil, Salmon fish, Avocado, Meat, Poultry, Nuts & Seeds. Avoid Saturated fats & Trans fats from diet.

4. Vitamins and Minerals:

- Vitamins and minerals are considered micronutrients vital for immune function, bone and eye health, and various metabolic functions of the body, as well as energy production.

- Different vitamins and minerals are responsible for different body functions and health. For example, viatmin C is essential for immunity and skin health, while vitamin D and calcium are essential for bone and heart health.

- Although all the vitamins and minerals are important for a healthy body, vitamin B12 and vitamin D are particularly vital for bodily metabolic functions.

How Vitamin B12 Deficiency Can Affect Your Health: A Real-Life Example:

A 37-year-old woman frequently experienced mouth ulcers that were often clotted with blood before bursting. When she consulted a physician, a Complete Blood Count (CBC) test revealed low levels of iron and hemoglobin. Her hemoglobin count was just 6, which is considered very low. The doctor explained that the mouth ulcers were a result of her anemia and prescribed iron and folic acid supplements to raise her hemoglobin levels to normal. However, after two months of taking these supplements, there was no improvement in her hemoglobin levels.

As her condition worsened, she sought help from a hematology specialist in an emergency. The specialist repeated the CBC test along with additional blood tests to investigate the cause of her persistent low hemoglobin and iron levels. Despite her long-term use of iron and folic acid supplements, her hemoglobin levels remained unchanged.

The hematology specialist then recommended a vitamin B12 test, which revealed that her vitamin B12 levels were significantly below the normal range. The doctor prescribed B12 supplements, and after two months of taking them, her hemoglobin levels improved and returned to normal. Additionally, her mouth ulcers and facial pimples disappeared.

This experience highlighted that her health issues, including anemia, mouth ulcers, pimples, and hair loss, were due to a vitamin B12 deficiency. With the appropriate treatment, she no longer faced these health problems.

A well-balanced diet helps provide the vitamins and minerals you need, and taking a daily multivitamin and mineral supplement can help ensure you get the proper amounts.

5. Phytonutrients:-

•   Phytonutrients are natural compounds produced by plant foods. They offer a number of benefits, such as preventing disease, enhancing immunity, and repairing DNA damage. Their pigments give fruits and vegetables their beautiful colors. That's why it's important to eat colorful, plant-based meals.

6. Fiber:-

•   Fiber is a crucial nutrient for the digestive process. It soothes the digestive tract and also helps to promote smooth bowel movements. It promotes the growth of good bacteria inside the digestive tract.

•   The best sources of dietary fiber are green vegetables, fruits, whole grains, and beans. Fiber is present in large quantities in the outer layer of green vegetables, fruits, and whole grains. The daily requirement of fiber for our body is 25 grams.

7. Water:-

•   Our body is made up of 70% water. Therefore, water is a vital part of a balanced diet. Without consuming an adequate quantity of water at proper intervals and maintaining correct hydration practices, our body cannot absorb nutrients properly.

• Water helps to hydrate our body, aids in digestion, transports nutrients to   different cells, regulates body temperature, and facilitates the easy excretion of waste. Water has zero calories.

• It plays a vital role during the weight loss process. Remember, The daily requirement of water is 8 glasses per day, with each glass being 8 ounces (240 ml). Drink water slowly, sip by sip, rather than quickly, so that it can be properly absorbed and aid digestion.

• Always drink water while sitting, not standing, as drinking water while standing may contribute to arthritis. Water can also lubricate different joints and tissues in the body. Never drink water during meals or within at least 1 hour of eating.

• A deficiency in water intake can lead to severe headaches, various gastrointestinal issues, and skin problems.

In my personal case, I was suffering from acute gastrointestinal issues like IBS (Irritable Bowel Syndrome) and also experienced various allergies and rashes on my skin. When I observed my lifestyle, I found that the quantity and manner of drinking water daily were not correct. Additionally, my sleep timing and pattern were off, and my daily diet was not balanced. After conducting various researches and receiving guidance from a wellness coach, I changed my lifestyle and sleep pattern, adjusted my water intake, and began eating balanced diets. This helped me achieve a new version of myself with no headaches, no digestive issues, and no skin allergies.

➢ **Practical Tips for Adopting a Balanced Diet:-**

We have already discussed the concept and importance of a balanced diet for holistic wellness above. Adopting a balanced diet can significantly enhance your overall well-being. Some practical tips are highlighted below to help you adopt a balanced diet in your daily routine effectively.

1) Plan Your Meals:-

• Plan your meals at least for a week or month considering your BMI and ideal weight. As the meal plan may differ according to a person's ideal weight goal (weight loss, weight gain, or weight maintenance), plan your personalized meal plan under the guidance of your nutritionist, wellness coach, or health practitioner. The benefit of making a meal plan is that you will avoid last-minute choices of unhealthy food.

• When planning your meals, consider the requirements of the key nutrients described above, the calorie value of food items, and another important parameter: the 'Glycemic Index' of food. The Glycemic Index (GI) is a scale of 0–100 that measures how much a food increases blood sugar levels. This means it ranks carbohydrate-containing foods based on the rate of their digestion and the increase in blood glucose levels over a certain period of time (generally 2 hours). So, choose low GI foods for a healthy body. Low GI foods help to minimize diabetes and to lose excess body fat.

• After preparing your meal plan, you can create a grocery list accordingly. The benefits of making a grocery list will help you purchase the right quality and quantity of food items more. In this way, you can avoid buying processed foods, which helps to maintain the concept of a balanced diet.

2) Portion Control:-

• The core objective of portion control is to guide individuals to choose a healthy amount of a certain food to get the requisite nutrients and avoid excess calorie intake from overeating. You may use the "Plate Method" to guide these portion sizes. Plates are available on the market with markings to help serve your food while maintaining proper portion sizes.

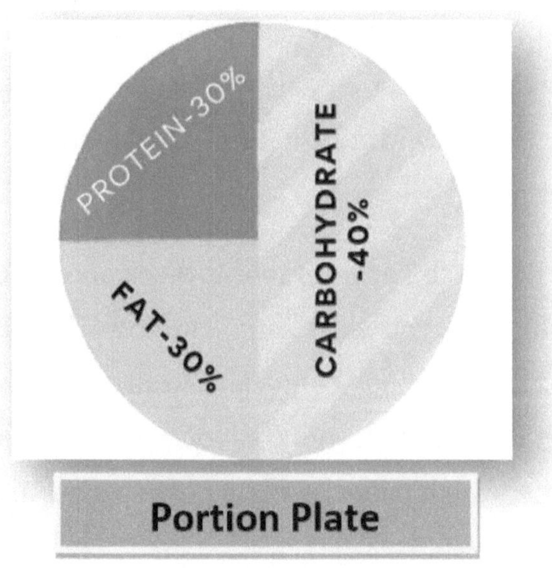

Portion Plate

- You can fill half of your plate with vegetables, one quarter with whole grains, and one quarter with lean protein. Use the "Plate Method" to guide portion sizes: fill half your plate with vegetables, one-quarter with whole grains, and one-quarter with lean protein. This visual guide helps in managing portion sizes and ensuring a balanced intake of nutrients.

- Each time, incorporate a variety of foods in the above proportions to maintain a diverse intake of nutrients and add variety to your meals. Eating a variety of colorful fruits and vegetables helps you get a range of vitamins and minerals.

- Practice mindful eating by paying attention to hunger and fullness signals from your body. It is best to apply the "20-Minute Rule" for eating to avoid overeating.

- Research suggests that it takes about 20 minutes from the time you start eating for your brain to signal the rest of your body (especially your stomach) that it's full. This is possible only if you eat slowly and enjoy each bite, which helps regulate portion sizes and prevent overeating.

- It is easier to catch the body's signals by eating mindfully, concentrating solely on your food and avoiding distractions from screens (TV or mobile).

3) Adopt Healthy Cooking Methods:

- During the preparation of your food, always adopt healthy cooking methods with a main focus on preserving the nutrients and making the food less caloric. You can use cooking methods such as steaming, grilling, and baking so that less oil or fat will be needed, making your food healthier and tastier. Nowadays, most nutritionists and health practitioners are suggesting and adopting zero-oil cooking methods because oil does not add taste; rather, spices do.

• You can use a variety of herbs (such as curry leaves, coriander leaves, bay leaves, rosemary, oregano, thyme, mint, parsley, chives) and spices (such as cloves, ginger, turmeric, coriander, black pepper) to add flavor and taste to your cooked food without extra calories or sodium. You can also use lemon juice to enhance the flavor of food without relying on high-fat sauces.

4) Incorporating Healthy Smart snacks :

• As per nutrition philosophy, it is found that adopting five meal plans can be considered balanced and healthy. Including three major meals (i.e., breakfast, lunch, and dinner), you can add two healthy and smart snacks between these major meals that combine protein and fiber to keep you full and energized.

• Good choices for healthy snacks are whole fruits like apple, berries, sprouts, a handful of soaked nuts, almond and different healthy seeds like flax seeds, pumpkin seeds, sunflower seeds, chia seeds, boiled eggs, steamed tofu, green vegetable salads and Greek yogurt with berries. These choices provide sustained energy and help maintain balanced nutrition between meals.

- Maintain a consistent time for all three major meals and two inter-meal snacks. You can schedule breakfast from 7 a.m. to 8 a.m., then have a small healthy snack between 10 a.m. and 11 a.m., lunch between 12 p.m. and 1 p.m., another small healthy snack between 4 p.m. and 5 p.m., and dinner between 7 p.m. and 8 p.m.

- Remember, portion control also applies to small snacks. Eat smaller quantities of snacks and use small containers to avoid overeating.

- The benefits of incorporating snacks into your meal plan include avoiding overeating by maintaining hunger control and balanced nutrition. This plays a major role in the weight loss process by reducing hunger and preventing overeating.

➤ What Science Says About the Benefits of a Balanced Diet:-

Research indicates that a balanced diet is another pillar of holistic health. It provides significant benefits, such as helping you achieve your ideal weight and protecting you from various chronic metabolic diseases like diabetes, thyroid disorders, high blood pressure, gastrointestinal disorders, cardiovascular diseases, and certain cancers. Here are some of the important benefits of a balanced diet according to scientific researchWhat Science Says About the Benefits of a Balanced Diet:

- **Weight Management:**

- A healthy weight (ideal weight) can be attained and maintained with balanced nutrition by providing the body with the right proportions of macronutrients and micronutrients while controlling calorie intake.

- Research highlights that diets with a proper balance of proteins, fats, and carbohydrates help regulate appetite and metabolism, making it easier to maintain a healthy weight (Johnston et al., 2014).

- **Digestive Health:**

- Research says that a high fiber diet helps to improve the Gut microbiota composition and reduces the risk of various gastrointestinal disorders such as bloating, GERD, constipation and colorectal cancer. (De Vries et al., 2016).

- Prebiotics & Probiotics are crucial nutrients to enhance the gut health by supporting a healthy balance of gut bacteria. It results the healthy digestive system and improvising a high immunity of the body. (Gibson et al., 2017).

- **Prevention of chronic metabolic diseases :**

- Research consistently shows that a balanced diet rich in fruits, vegetables, whole grains, and lean proteins helps to lower the risk of cardiovascular diseases. Studies like the PREDIMED trial have demonstrated that this dietary pattern improves heart health and reduces mortality (Estruch et al., 2013).

- A diet of low G.I foods having high in fiber low in saturated fats can improve insulin sensitivity and reduce the risk of type 2 diabetes. (Slavin, 2013).

➢ **Conclusion:-**

It is understood that Balanced Diet plays a crucial role in holistic wellness; it helps to attain ideal body weight, prevention of chronic metabolic diseases. The intention of balanced diet is to consumption of nutrient dense and low caloric food.

It is a important proverb that 'Food is Medicine', so take the responsibility of your own body and give the importance on your daily food you eat otherwise medicine will become your food. So, to prevent yourself from illness and get holistic wellness, plan your balanced diet taking into consideration above discussed tips and information under the guidance of any wellness coach or dietician or any health practitioner.

But achieving holistic health requires more than just balanced nutrition. Another essential component is proper rest and recovery. In the next chapter, we will explore the importance of sleep patterns and how quality sleep is vital for restoring your body, enhancing your cognitive function, and ensuring long-term health and wellness.

"Let food be thy medicine and medicine be thy food."

- Hippocrates

<u>Key Take Aways</u>:-

❖ The food we eat is not just intended to satisfy our hunger; rather, it should provide all the nutrients required for our body on a daily basis to remain healthy and active.

❖ The basic concept of a balanced diet is to consume nutrient-dense and lower-calorie foods. Our daily diet should be balanced, meaning it should consist of macronutrients, micronutrients, and phytonutrients.

❖ The prime intention is to ensure that every meal contributes to our overall health and wellness by providing essential nutrients with fewer calories. A balanced diet supports the body's metabolic functions, promotes energy, and helps prevent various chronic diseases.

❖ According to the concept of Global Nutrition Philosophy, our body needs a daily balanced diet comprising 40% carbohydrates, 30% healthy fats, 30% protein, and 25 grams of fiber.

❖ Protein is essential for building and repairing tissues, including muscles, and is important for immune function and the production of enzymes and hormones.

❖ Carbohydrates are the body's primary source of energy. Dietary Fats support heart, brain and joint health, as well as cell functions.

❖ Vitamins and Minerals are considered micronutrients vital for immune function, bone and eye health, and various metabolic functions of the body.

❖ Fiber is the most important nutrient for the digestive process. It soothes the digestive tract and helps promote smooth bowel movements. It also promotes the growth of good bacteria in the digestive tract.

❖ Water helps to hydrate our body, aids in digestion, transports nutrients to different cells, regulates body temperature, and facilitates the easy excretion of waste. Water has zero calories.

❖ Plan your personalized meal under the guidance of your nutritionist, wellness coach, or health practitioner.

❖ You can fill half of your plate with vegetables, one quarter with whole grains and one quarter with lean protein.

❖ Eating a variety of colorful fruits and vegetables helps you get range of vitamins & minerals.

❖ Practice mindful eating by paying attention to hunger and fullness signals from your body. It is best to apply the "20-minute rule" for eating to avoid overeating.

❖ You can use cooking methods such as steaming, grilling, and baking so that less oil or fat will be needed, making your food healthier and tastier.

❖ Include three major meals (i.e., breakfast, lunch, and dinner), and add two healthy and smart snacks between these major meals that combine protein and fiber to keep you full and energized.

❖ Research highlights that diets with a proper balance of proteins, fats, and carbohydrates help regulate appetite and metabolism, making it easier to maintain a healthy weight.

❖ Research consistently shows that a balanced diet rich in fruits, vegetables, whole grains, and lean proteins helps lower the risk of cardiovascular diseases and type2 diabetes.

Chapter 3

Sleep Patterns and Wellness

"Sleep is the single most effective thing we can do to reset our brain and body health each day"

- Dr Matthew Walker

➢ **Introduction:-**

In order to maintain overall wellness, physical health, and mental health, relaxation and sleep are essential. We spend about a third of our lives asleep. Sleep is crucial and automatic, without which our body can't function well. It's just as important as eating, drinking, and breathing. Sleep is vital for both our mental and physical health. It helps to heal and refresh not only our bodies but also our brains.

Our sleep pattern is an indicator of the circadian rhythm. The circadian rhythm is the internal biological clock of your body that controls the 24 hours cycle of different biological processes including sleep and wake patterns of your body. The control center responsible for the circadian rhythm is located in the hypothalamus of the brain. It is synchronized to the outside world by light and darkness, while it is synchronized to other parts of the body by the timing of when we eat.

Sleep is the most profound predictor of a healthy circadian rhythm. When we disturb our sleep, it affects not only our physical health but also brain health. Research has shown that chronically sleep-deprived animals and humans have weaker immune systems, less resistance to even mild infections and viruses, and face more health challenges or even death. Therefore, maintaining a consistent sleep schedule is a key strategy for maintaining better immunity.

➢ **The Importance of Quality Sleep for Physical and Mental Well-being:-**

In order to maintain overall wellness, physical health, and mental health, sleep is essential. It promotes physical revival, stress reduction, brain health, emotional control, productivity, and a higher standard of living. *Here is why quality sleep is important for physical and mental health.*

A] For Physical Health:-

- By maintaining quality sleep or deep sleep, your body immunity increases and also helps in the production of growth hormones in the body.

- During deep sleep your body repairs the tissues, muscles and bones.

- Quality sleep helps to regulate hormones that control your hunger and appetite. In contrast, poor sleep will interrupt these hormones resulting in weight gain and a high risk of various metabolic disorders.

- Maintaining proper timing and duration of sleep helps to control the blood pressure and stress levels resulting in a reduced risk of cardiovascular disease.

- Quality sleep can enhance the skin radiance. Additionally, good sleep can boost your energy level and result in improved performance output.

B] For Mental Health:-

- During sleep, our brain processes the information we've taken in, strengthens our memories, and performs important maintenance tasks. This helps us function better during the day.

- Quality sleep can improve your focus, attention, patience and enhance your quick decision- making ability.

- Quality sleep can increase cheerfulness and alertness in all activities.

- Maintaining a good sleep pattern can reduce our stress levels and make us more relaxed, resulting in improved brain performance.

- With quality sleep, our brain can release more happy hormones , such as endorphins.

Individuals can improve their general health, mental health, and attain a sense of holistic well-being by valuing and giving priority to quality sleep. Additionally, due to a good sleep pattern, individuals can experience a better life, improved work performance, good behavior patterns, and a healthy physiology.

➢ **Best Tips for Improving Sleep Pattern:-**

After recognizing the importance of quality sleep for both physical and mental health, it's time to focus on some tips for improving your sleep pattern for effective results in your body.

• Research says that babies and toddlers may sleep as much as 12 hours each day; children and teenagers should spend nine hours in bed; and adults should try to be in bed for eight hours.

• Maintaining a consistent sleep schedule is a powerful strategy to maintain better immunity. A Sleep schedule involves maintaining a particular time for being awake and going to bed, which can strengthen the circadian rhythm.

• For a sound and quality sleep, it is better to complete your dinner at least 2 to 3 hours before sleep and drink less water in the hour or two before bed to reduce the chances of needing to get up during the night to use the bathroom. This can help improve sleep quality and prevent disruptions.

• However, it is recommended to stay hydrated throughout the day and to drink less water at night before sleep. If you find yourself frequently needing to wake up at night, you might need to look at other factors that could be affecting your sleep and consult a health practitioner.

• Changing the ambiance of the bedroom can have a positive impact on achieving sound sleep. You can dim your bedroom light for two to three hours before bedtime.

• You may find it helpful to use an aromatic room freshener with calming scents and play slow, soothing music in your bedroom to create a relaxing environment that supports better sleep.

• Adding simple activities to your nightly routine, such as taking a bath and brushing your teeth, can have a positive impact on your sleep quality.

• Avoid eating high-calorie, oily foods at dinner. Instead, opt for easily digestible, steamed, or low-oil foods. This can contribute to a better night's sleep. As discussed in the previous chapter, high-calorie foods can affect your gut, which in turn affects your mind.

• Limit your daily screen time and avoid using screens for at least one hour before bedtime. Research indicates that screen use at night can disrupt sleep quality.

• Engage in physical exercise and pranayama (breathing exercises) daily for at least 30-45 minutes to help you relax and feel refreshed, which can contribute to better sleep quality at night.

• Maintaining a consistent sleep schedule—going to bed and waking up at the same time each day—not only improves the quality of your sleep but also promotes overall health. Waking up early is particularly beneficial, as research suggests that the air contains higher levels of oxygen before sunrise, which can help you feel more refreshed.

• Avoid overthinking and focus on living in the present moment, or the 'NOW Zone,' to achieve better sleep quality. 'NOW' stands for 'No Overwhelming Worries.' Staying relaxed and present can help you get a more restful night's sleep."

• Practice mindfulness meditation for at least 15-30 minutes daily to bring calmness to your mind and promote relaxation, which can help improve the quality of your sleep.

➢ **Research and Personal Insights on the Benefits of Sleep Patterns:**

Before delving into the research on how sleep patterns benefit our wellness, I'd like to share my personal story of how adjusting my own sleep routine helped me achieve my health goals.

My Journey from Night Owl to Early Bird: A Personal Transformation:-

Growing up, I was always a night owl. My school years were marked by late-night study sessions, and I would wake up only when the morning was well underway. I had never seen a sunrise and believed that waking up early was simply impossible for me. Staying up late felt exciting and productive, especially since my hostel environment during higher studies reinforced my late-night habits.

However, these habits started taking a toll on my health. Over time, I began to experience severe acidity and digestive issues. My gut health deteriorated, and I frequently had mucus in my stool. Persistent headaches and vomiting became regular parts of my life. Despite frequent visits to family doctors, my condition didn't improve.

Realizing that medication alone wasn't solving my problems, I turned to books and online resources for advice on achieving true wellness. During this period, I was deeply inspired by my beloved father, who had always emphasized the importance of a healthy lifestyle. He often spoke about the benefits of going to bed early and rising with the sun. Motivated by his wisdom, I came to understand that I needed to make more than just temporary fixes; I needed to commit to lasting changes in my diet and sleep patterns. With this inspiration from my father, I sought guidance from a wellness coach and embarked on a transformative journey to overhaul my sleep routine. Now, as I write this, I cherish his memory and the impact his advice had on my path to better health.

I set a new goal: to shift my sleep schedule to align with a healthier lifestyle. I committed to going to bed by 10 P.M. and waking up at 4:30 A.M. The initial transition was tough, but I gave myself a 21-day challenge to stick with this new routine. I followed every tip for quality sleep and made sure to adjust my diet as well.

Gradually, the change brought remarkable results. I started to wake up feeling refreshed, energized, and ready to embrace the beauty and tranquility of the early morning. My days became more productive, and I felt a newfound sense of vitality. My gut health improved, my headaches diminished, and I felt more relaxed overall.

Now, I am proud to say that I've transformed from a night owl into an early bird. This shift has brought me a healthier, more active lifestyle. I'm grateful for this change and the holistic well-being it has brought into my life. My story serves as a testament to the profound benefits of adopting a balanced sleep pattern and a positive mindset. It's a reminder that with determination and the right approach, we can all achieve better health and happiness.

Now, here to find some of the researches regarding the benefit of the sleep pattern.

➢ *Effects of Sleep Patterns on Gut Microbiome*

Recent research has highlighted the crucial role sleep and circadian rhythms play in maintaining our metabolic health. Studies, including those conducted by Dana Withrow, Samuel J. Bowers, Christopher M.

Depner, Antonio Gonzalez, Amy C. Reynolds, and Kenneth P. Wright, Jr., have explored how poor sleep and disrupted circadian rhythms can negatively impact our metabolism.

When we don't get enough sleep or our sleep patterns are out of sync with our natural body clock, it affects the diversity and function of the gut microbiome—the community of microbes living in our intestines. These changes can alter the production of important metabolites, like short-chain fatty acids and bile acids. These substances are involved in various bodily functions, including inflammation, energy balance, and hormone regulation.

The research reviewed mainly from the past two years suggests that these disruptions in the gut microbiome might be a key reason why lack of sleep and circadian misalignment lead to metabolic problems. Essentially, the gut microbiome could be a link between poor sleep and metabolic issues.

For more detailed insights, refer to the study by Withrow et al., which explores these connections in both human and animal models and supports the idea that a healthy sleep pattern is vital for maintaining a balanced gut microbiome and overall metabolic health.

Source: Withrow, D., Bowers, S. J., Depner, C. M., González, A., Reynolds, A. C., & Wright, K. P., Jr. (2024). Sleep and Circadian Disruption and the Gut Microbiome—Possible Links to Dysregulated Metabolism.

➢ *Sleep Behaviors and Their Impact on the Progression from Pre-Diabetes to Type 2 Diabetes Mellitus*

• *Recent research has investigated how different sleep behaviors and related habits affect the progression from pre-diabetes to type 2 diabetes mellitus (T2DM) in adults by Samiul A Mostafa, Sandra Campos Mena, Christina Antza, George Balanos, Krishnarajah Nirantharakumar, and Abd A Tahrani. A comprehensive review and meta-analysis on this topic reveal several key findings:*

• *The research highlights a clear link between getting insufficient sleep and an increased risk of advancing from pre-diabetes to T2DM. People who don't get enough sleep are more likely to develop full-blown diabetes.*

• *Although the data is limited, there are indications that insomnia and working night shifts may also be associated with a higher risk of progressing to T2DM. However, more studies are needed to better understand these connections.*

➢ *The review suggests that exploring various sleep disorders and their interactions is crucial for understanding how they contribute to the development of T2DM. Adjusting specific sleep behaviors could potentially help in preventing the progression from pre-diabetes to T2DM.*

• *Overall, this research underscores the importance of considering sleep patterns as a factor in diabetes prevention strategies, alongside other lifestyle changes.*

Source:- Samiul A Mostafa, Sandra Campos Mena, Christina Antza, George Balanos, Krishnarajah Nirantharakumar, and Abd A Tahrani-Sleep behaviours and associated habits and the progression of pre-diabetes to type 2 diabetes mellitus in adults: A systematic review and meta-analysis

> **Emotional Regulation and Sleep**

In a 2007 study by Matthew Walker and his team, published in the journal Neuropsychopharmacology, researchers looked at how sleep impacts our emotions. They found that getting enough sleep is crucial for managing our emotions, mainly because it affects the amygdala, a part of the brain that processes feelings. People who slept well were better at handling emotions and didn't react as strongly to negative situations.

This study matches my own experience. Since I started improving my sleep habits, I've noticed that I feel less emotional and stressed. Walker's research backs this up, showing that good sleep is key to keeping our emotions stable.

If you're interested in reading the study, you can find it here: Walker, M., & Stickgold, A. (2007). Sleep and emotional regulation: The role of the amygdala. Neuropsychopharmacology.

Retrieved from
https://www.nature.com/articles/sj.npp.1301242.

➤ Sleep is essential to health: an American Academy of Sleep Medicine position statement

Recent research has investigated how sleep is essential to health by Ramar K, Malhotra RK, Carden KA, et al.

Sleep is crucial for our health, and not getting enough of it or having sleep problems can harm our well-being and safety. The Healthy People 2030 initiative aims to improve our health, productivity, and quality of life by promoting better sleep. This includes not just getting enough sleep, but also ensuring it is good quality, happens at the right times, is regular, and free from disorders.

The American Academy of Sleep Medicine (AASM) stresses that sleep is vital for health. They believe that more focus should be put on sleep in education, healthcare, long-term care, public health efforts, and workplaces. More research is needed to understand how important sleep is for public health and how lack of sleep contributes to health inequalities.

Source: Ramar K, Malhotra RK, Carden KA, et al. Sleep is essential to health: an American Academy of

Sleep Medicine position statement. J Clin Sleep Med. 2021;17(10):2115

> **Understanding Sleep Extension and Its Effects on Cardio metabolic Health: Mechanisms and Practical Insights**

Recent research has investigated how Sleep Extension affect the Cardiometabolic by Kara M. Duraccio, Sarah Kamhout, Kelly G. Baron, Sirimon Reutrakul, Christopher M. Depner

Short sleep duration is linked to a higher risk of cardiometabolic diseases and has become a widespread issue affecting children, teens, and adults. The reasons behind this connection are complex and involve disruptions in circadian rhythms, eating habits, appetite hormones, brain areas related to pleasure-driven eating, physical activity, changes in gut bacteria, and reduced insulin sensitivity.

Increasing sleep duration, known as sleep extension, is a promising approach to understanding and potentially reducing the risk of these diseases. If proven effective, extending sleep could improve cardiometabolic health throughout life. Current research indicates that sleep extension is possible and might offer health benefits, but there are challenges. Most studies are short-term (2–8 weeks), use different methods for extending sleep, and examine a range of health outcomes, often with small sample sizes, which limits strong conclusions.

To address these issues, we need larger, long-term studies with well-defined methods and participants who habitually sleep poorly and have cardiometabolic risks. Comparing different sleep extension techniques through randomized controlled trials will help identify the most effective strategies. Ongoing and future research should focus on the potential benefits of sleep extension to improve health and quality of life for those struggling with short sleep.

Source:- Kara M. Duraccio, Sarah Kamhout, Kelly G. Baron, Sirimon Reutrakul, Christopher M. Depner- Sleep extension and cardiometabolic health: what it is, possible mechanisms and real-world applications

➢ Conclusion:-

Based on the above discussed topic, along with personal experiences and recent research findings, it's clear that our sleep patterns play a vital role in our overall health. Quality sleep affects not just our physical health but also our mental and emotional health. By implementing the proven tips and strategies outlined in this chapter, you can significantly improve your sleep and enhance your holistic health.

In the next chapter, we will explore the importance of exercise and its profound effects on our overall wellness. Understanding how physical activity complements good sleep can further boost your health and quality of life Stay tuned and continue applying these insights to lead a balanced and healthier life.

<u>Key Take Aways:</u>

❖ Sleep is vital for both our mental and physical health.

❖ Research has shown that chronically sleep-deprived animals and humans have weaker immune systems.

❖ During deep sleep your body repairs the tissues, muscles and bones.

❖ Quality sleep helps to regulate hormones that control your hunger and appetite.

❖ It helps to control blood pressure and reduces the risk of cardiovascular diseases.

❖ It enhance our decision taking ability, brain functioning.

❖ Maintaining a consistent sleep schedule is a powerful strategy to maintain better immunity.

❖ Limit your daily screen time and avoid using screens for at least one hour before bedtime.

❖ Avoid over thinking and focus on living in the present moment, or the 'NOW Zone,' to achieve better sleep quality.

❖ For a sound & quality sleep, it is better to complete your dinner at least 2 to 3 hours before sleep and drink less water in the hour or two before bed.

❖ Changing the aura of the bedroom can have a positive impact on achieving sound sleep.

❖ Research says that not having enough quality sleep, the diversity and functions of Gut Microbiome got affected and then consequently the immunity.

❖   The research highlights a clear link between getting insufficient sleep and an increased risk of advancing from pre-diabetes to T2DM (Type 2 Diabetes Mellitus).

❖   Research finds out that Short sleep duration is linked to a higher risk of cardiometabolic diseases.

CHAPTER 4

EXERCISE FOR VITALITY

"Push harder than yesterday if you want a different tomorrow."

– Vincent Williams Sr.

➤ **A Father's Legacy: Revitalizing My Health Through Exercise:**

My journey to a healthier lifestyle was profoundly influenced by a combination of personal struggles and the unwavering support of my father. In my earlier years, my life was marked by unhealthy habits: late nights, oversleeping, and a general disinterest in exercise. My health took a turn when I was diagnosed with acute sinusitis at a young age. My ENT specialist advised me that regular exercise could help manage and potentially cure my condition once I turned 18. Despite this advice, I struggled with my sleep patterns and remained reliant on medication, showing little interest in adopting a healthier routine.

Throughout this period, my father was a constant source of motivation. He encouraged me to wake up early and dedicate at least 30 minutes a day to exercise. He believed, and demonstrated through his own life, that consistent physical activity could lead to better health and alleviate my sinusitis and IBS symptoms. His own daily routine included walking 6 to 7 kilometers in a medicinal plantation park and practicing yoga. His commitment to fitness was evident; he was never afflicted by chronic diseases and appeared to be in perfect health.

Inspired by his example and motivated by the promising health benefits of exercise that I encountered through various sources, I decided to embrace a consistent exercise routine of 30 to 45 minutes daily. This decision led to remarkable changes: my sleep pattern improved, I began waking up earlier, and I experienced a surge of energy and vitality throughout the day. My sinusitis symptoms and gut health issues significantly improved, and I found myself less dependent on medication. Additionally, I achieved and maintained my ideal weight.

Writing this chapter brings an emotional weight, as my beloved father, who was the driving force behind my lifestyle transformation, is no longer with me. Tragically, he passed away in an unexpected road accident while heading to his morning walk. I miss him deeply. His daily motivation and example were crucial in helping me achieve better health and well-being.

If my story inspires you to adopt a healthier lifestyle and commit to daily exercise, it would be the greatest tribute to my father. His legacy lives on through the positive changes he helped me make, and I hope his story can inspire others to embrace the transformative power of exercise.

Let's start by exploring the science behind how exercise can enhance energy levels and reduce fatigue. We'll look at the physiological mechanisms at play and how adopting a routine of physical activity can significantly impact your health, just as it did for me.

From understanding how exercise helps to alleviate symptoms of chronic conditions to integrating it into your daily life, this chapter will guide you through the transformative power of movement.

➤ **The Science Behind Exercise and Energy: How Physical Activity Boosts Energy Levels and Reduces Fatigue:-**

In a comprehensive review by Darren E.R. Warburton, Crystal Whitney Nicol, and Shannon S.D. Bredin titled "Health benefits of physical activity: the evidence"

published in PMC, we examined how not getting enough exercise can lead to serious health problems and even shorten your life.

The evidence is clear: regular physical activity is incredibly important for preventing and managing a wide range of chronic diseases, such as heart disease, diabetes, cancer (including breast and colon cancer), high blood pressure, obesity, depression, and osteoporosis.

The review also highlights that following the physical activity guidelines provided by Health Canada can make a significant difference, especially for those who have been inactive. Simply increasing your activity level can lead to substantial health improvements.

The connection between exercise and better health is strong and straightforward. The more active you are, the better your overall health tends to be.

Lack of exercise is a major risk factor for many health issues, including heart disease, diabetes, certain cancers, obesity, high blood pressure, bone and joint problems, and depression. In fact, more Canadians are inactive than those with other modifiable risk factors.

This review brings together the latest evidence on how exercise can help prevent early death and various diseases. It also discusses how different levels and types of exercise impact your health.

Previous reviews have covered similar ground, but this review highlights key studies and new discoveries about how physical activity improves health and reduces the risk of chronic diseases.

Research shows that not getting enough exercise is a major risk factor for chronic health challenges. Studies confirm that adhering to physical activity guidelines, like those from Health Canada, can significantly enhance your health.

By increasing your activity levels, you can reduce your risk of these diseases, which in turn helps to boost your energy levels and combat fatigue.

This means that regular physical activity not only helps prevent serious health conditions but also plays a vital role in enhancing your overall energy and reducing feelings of tiredness.

Incorporating exercise into your daily routine can lead to substantial improvements in how you feel on a day-to-day basis, making you more energetic and less prone to fatigue

Exercise also benefits your digestive system. **According to the Journal of the International Society of Sports Nutrition, regular physical activity helps maintain a healthy gut by increasing the variety of good bacteria and improving overall gut health.**

> **Types of Exercises and its Benefits:-**

Taking a balanced approach, in my opinion, is the best approach to living a healthy, active lifestyle. As per Global Nutrition Philosophy, 20% exercise is required to become holistically healthy.

1. Aerobic (Cardio) Exercise:

• Doing cardio exercises is great for your heart and helps burn extra calories. Since your heart is a muscle, working it out a few times a week can boost its performance.

• Regular cardio can also lower your resting heart rate, benefiting your long-term health. Examples of Cardio Exercise include walking, running, cycling, dancing, and swimming. As per WHO recommendation you can do at least 150 mins of moderate cardio exercise or at least 75 mins of intense cardio exercise each week.

• Cardio Exercise can give so much health benefits like it improves heart health. Strengthen the efficiency of your lungs.

• It helps in loosing unwanted fat and managing ideal weight by burning extra calories.

• It helps to release endorphins hormone than can improve your mood and reduce stress.

2. Resistance Exercise

- Resistance Exercise is also called strength training. It involves excercises designed to improve strength by working against a force.

- The primary benefits of resistance exercise include increased muscle strength, improved bone density, enhanced metabolic rate, and better overall functional fitness.

- Examples of Resistance excercises include weight lifting, push-ups, squats, and etc.

- It helps to boost your metabolism by burning more calories even at rest.

- It strengthens the bones by improving bone density.

3. Stretching Excercise

- Stretching exercises are movements designed to improve flexibility and range of motion in your muscles and joints. They help to lengthen and relax muscles, which can enhance overall mobility, reduce muscle tension.

- Different examples of stretching exercises are Yoga, static stretching.

- They improves the mobility and flexibility of your joints and muscles.

- They can improve overall posture and alignment.

- They helps to reduce muscle tension and stress.

4. High-Intensity Interval Training (HIIT)

- High-Intensity Interval Training (HIIT) is a form of exercise that alternates between short, intense bursts of activity and periods of lower-intensity exercise or rest.

- The structure of HIIT workouts is flexible, which allows you to tailor them to your fitness level and goals.

- Examples of HIIT include short bursts of intense exercise followed by rest (e.g., sprinting followed by walking)

- HIIT workouts can be shorter in duration but still highly effective, making them a good option for people with busy schedules.

- The intense bursts can enhance heart and lung health.

- HIIT can elevate your metabolism for hours after the workout, leading to more calories burned.

5. Breathing Exercises:

- Breathing exercises are techniques designed to improve your breathing efficiency, lung capacity, and overall respiratory health. They involve practicing specific patterns of inhalation and exhalation to enhance your physical and mental well-being.

- There are various types of breathing excercises such as:

- Abdominal breathing for relaxation, improving lung function, and enhancing oxygen delivery to different parts of the body.

- Square breathing: Inhale through your nose for a count of four, hold your breath for a count of four, exhale through your mouth for a count of four, and then hold your breath again for a count of four before starting the cycle over.

- Alternate Nostril Breathing (Nadi Shodhana) by Use your thumb to close one nostril and inhale deeply through the open nostril. Close the open nostril with your ring finger, release the thumb to open the other nostril, and exhale through it. Inhale through the same nostril, then switch and exhale through the other nostril.

- Alternate Nostril Breathing (Nadi Shodhana): **Use** your thumb to close one nostril and inhale deeply through the open nostril. Close the open nostril with your ring finger, release the thumb to open the other nostril, and exhale through it. Inhale through the same nostril, then switch and exhale through the other nostril.

- The 4-7-8 Breathing technique can be done by inhaling through your nose for a count of four, holding your breath for a count of seven, and then exhaling slowly through your mouth for a count of eight.

- 4-7-8 Breathing helps with relaxation, improves sleep, and reduces anxiety.

- Breathing exercises can be practiced independently or integrated into other activities like yoga, meditation, or even during exercise routines.

- They Promote relaxation and helps manage stress levels.

6. Recreational Activities

- Our regular activities like playing sports, gardening, doing any activities like washing clothes , and cleaning the home without using any gadgets, can be considered as a type of exercise.

- It makes exercise fun.

- It enhances socialization and engagement with others.

Incorporating a mix of these exercises into your routine can offer comprehensive health benefits and keep your workouts varied and engaging. An exercise plan is very important for a weight loss program , as well as for your health and vitality .

➢ How Does Exercise Help in Balancing Your Hormones?

In today's busy world, spending time outdoors can be incredibly refreshing and beneficial for both your body and mind. Taking a break from technology and immersing yourself in nature helps to reset and rejuvenate your brain.

Exercise influences a wide range of hormones in the body, each playing a critical role in maintaining health and well-being. Here's how various hormones are affected by physical activity:

- **Cortisol:**

Often referred to as the stress hormone, cortisol is released in response to physical and psychological stress.

Regular moderate exercise can help regulate cortisol levels, preventing chronic elevation that is linked to negative health outcomes such as weight gain, high blood pressure, cardiovascular disease and impaired immune function.

High cortisol levels can negatively impact thyroid function and hormone balance, so reducing stress through exercise supports thyroid health.

- **Adrenaline (Epinephrine):**

This hormone is released during exercise to increase heart rate, blood flow to muscles, and energy availability. Exercise stimulates adrenaline production, which helps improve physical performance and energy levels.

- **Endorphins**:

Cardio exercise boosts the production of endorphins, the brain's feel-good chemicals. Endorphins are natural painkillers produced by the brain during exercise. They help enhance mood and create a sense of well-being, often referred to as the "runner's high.

It can also be experienced through activities like playing tennis, badminton or even walking. Cardio workouts can provide a sense of meditation in motion—by focusing on your exercise, you can lower your stress levels.

As a result, even though you might feel physically tired afterward, you'll likely feel mentally refreshed. The increase in endorphins and other neurotransmitters during exercise contributes to an improved mood and a reduction in symptoms of depression and anxiety.

- **Insulin**:

Exercise helps manage insulin levels by reducing inflammation, which is important for diabetes control. Inflammation markers like IL-6 and CRP are linked to insulin resistance and diabetes. Regular exercise lowers these inflammatory markers and increases anti-inflammatory substances in the body.

By boosting anti-inflammatory cytokines and reducing harmful ones, exercise helps improve insulin sensitivity. It also lowers leptin levels and improves blood vessel function. Overall, staying active helps keep insulin levels in check and lowers the risk of diabetes.

Improved insulin sensitivity and hormonal balance support better metabolic function, aiding in weight management, reducing the risk of chronic diseases, and enhancing overall vitality.

- **Thyroid:-**

Regular exercise can help maintain a healthy metabolic rate by supporting the production and function of thyroid hormones. It can enhance T3 activity, which improves metabolism and energy levels.

Physical activity promotes healthy thyroid function by improving blood flow and reducing inflammation. This can help ensure that the thyroid gland functions efficiently.

Regular exercise can enhance the conversion of T4 (inactive thyroid hormone) to T3 (active thyroid hormone), which is crucial for regulating metabolism and energy.

It's important to avoid excessive or very high-intensity exercise, as it can increase cortisol levels and potentially impact thyroid health negatively.

- **Androgens:-**

Androgens are often elevated in women having PCOS issue. These are "male hormones and when their levels are elevated, can cause symptoms like acne, excessive hair growth, and scalp hair thinning. Reducing androgen levels can help alleviate these symptoms. Research indicates that resistance or strength training may improve androgen levels.

- **Progesterone:-**

In PCOS, the ovaries may not release an egg (ovulate) regularly, leading to low levels of progesterone. This hormonal imbalance contributes to irregular menstrual cycles and can affect the uterine lining.Moderate-intensity resistance training and cardio exercise can help to balance progesterone levels

- **Growth Hormone**:

Produced by the pituitary gland, growth hormone is essential for muscle growth, repair, and overall body composition. Exercise, particularly strength training and high-intensity interval training (HIIT), stimulates the release of growth hormone, contributing to muscle development and fat loss.

The above facts confirm that with the help of doing different exercises daily you can balance your different hormone levels to maintain your health and vitality.

➢ **Conclusion:-**

Based on the discussion, personal stories, and research findings, it's clear that exercise plays a vital role in our overall health. Regular physical activity is crucial for preventing and managing a wide range of chronic diseases.

We've explored different types of exercises and their specific benefits, emphasizing the importance of creating a personalized exercise plan tailored to your individual needs. Through this, we've seen how exercise can help balance hormone levels and contribute to holistic health and vitality.

According to the Global Nutrition philosophy, which was discussed in the previous chapter, achieving a healthy body requires a balance of 80% nutrition and 20% exercise. By integrating the insights gained from this chapter, you can better appreciate the role of exercise in this balance and make informed decisions about your personal health and fitness plan.

Key Take Aways:

❖ Research indicates that not getting enough exercise can lead to serious health problems and even shorten your life.

❖ Simply increasing your activity level can lead to substantial health improvements.

❖ Lack of exercise is a major risk factor for many health issues, including heart disease, diabetes, certain cancers, obesity, high blood pressure, bone and joint problems, and depression.

❖ Regular physical activity helps maintain a healthy gut by increasing the variety of good bacteria and improving overall gut health.

❖ According to WHO recommendations, you can do at least 150 minutes of moderate cardio exercise or at least 75 minutes of intense cardio exercise each week.

❖ Preparing an exercise plan by incorporating a mix of various exercises is very important for a weight loss program, as well as for your health and vitality.

❖ Exercise influences a wide range of hormones in the body, each playing a critical role in maintaining health and well-being.

❖ Physical activity promotes healthy thyroid function by improving blood flow and reducing inflammation.

❖ Endorphins are natural painkillers produced by the brain during exercise.

❖ Strength training and high-intensity interval training (HIIT), stimulate the release of growth hormone, contributing to muscle development and fat loss.

❖ Regular moderate exercise can help regulate cortisol levels, preventing chronic elevation that is linked to negative health outcomes.

❖ Resistance exercise helps to boost your metabolism by burning more calories even at rest and it strengthens bones by improving the bone density.

BIBLIOGRAPHY

✓ Insufficient sleep and circadian misalignment are associated with adverse metabolic health outcomes.

✓ *Withrow, D., Bowers, S. J., Depner, C. M., González, A., Reynolds, A. C., & Wright, K. P., Jr. (2024). Sleep and Circadian Disruption and the Gut Microbiome—Possible Links to Dysregulated Metabolism.*

✓ *Samiul A Mostafa, Sandra Campos Mena, Christina Antza, George Balanos, Krishna rajah, and Abd A Tahrani-Sleep behaviours and associated habits and the progression of pre-diabetes to type 2 diabetes mellitus in adults: A systematic review and meta-analysis*

✓ *Walker, M., & Stickgold, A. (2007). Sleep and emotional regulation: The role of the amygdala. Neuropsychopharmacology. Retrieved from https://www.nature.com/articles/sj.npp.1301242.*

✓ *Ramar K, Malhotra RK, Carden KA, et al. Sleep is essential to health: an American Academy of Sleep Medicine position statement. J Clin Sleep Med. 2021;17(10):2115*

✓ *Kara M. Duraccio, Sarah Kamhout, Kelly G. Baron, Sirimon Reutrakul, Christopher M. Depner- Sleep extension and cardiometabolic health: what it is, possible mechanisms and real-world applications*

- *comprehensive review by Darren E.R. Warburton, Crystal Whitney Nicol, and Shannon S.D. Bredin titled "Health benefits of physical activity: the evidence" published in PMC*

- *A diet of low G.I foods having high in fiber low in saturated fats can improve insulin sensitivity and reduce the risk of type 2 diabetes. (Slavin, 2013).*

- *high fiber diet helps to improve the Gut microbiota composition and reduces the risk of various gastrointestinal disorders such as bloating, GERD, constipation and colorectal cancer. (De Vries et al., 2016)*

- *Sleep and Circadian Disruption and the Gut MicrobiomePossible Links to Dysregulated Metabolism Published online 2020 Nov 28. doi: 10.1016/j.coemr.2020.11.009*

- *Ramar K, Malhotra RK, Carden KA, et al. Sleep is essential to health: an American Academy of Sleep Medicine position statement. J Clin Sleep Med. 2021;17(10):2115– 2119.*

- *Eat, Train, Sleep—Retreat? Hormonal Interactions of Intermittent Fasting, Exercise and Circadian Rhythm Published online 2021 Mar 30. doi: 10.3390/biom11040516*

- *Obesity Statistics In 2024 – Forbes Health website:- forbes.com/health/weight-loss/obesity-statistics*

- *Health benefits of physical activity: the evidence CMAJ. 2006 Mar 14; 174(6): 801–809 https://www.ncbi.nlm.nih.gov/pmc/articles/PMC1402378/*

- ✓ *Health Benefits of Hiking and Exercising Outdoors David Heber, Chairman, Herbalife Nutrition Institute January 23, 2024*

- ✓ *Human body weight - Wikipedia en.wikipedia.org/wiki/Human_body_weight*

- ✓ *https://www.worldobesity.org/resources/resource-library/world-obesity-atlas-2022*

- ✓ *https://www.who.int/health-topics/obesity*

- ✓ *10th edition of the IDF Diabetes Atlas reports https://idf.org/news/one-billion-people-globally-estimated-to-be-living-with-obesity-by-2030/*

About The Author

Rabi Narayan Mohanty is a wellness coach with a deep passion for health, fitness, and holistic living. Drawing from personal experience, Rabi Narayan has transformed a life once burdened by chronic health challenges into one of vitality and balance. After overcoming years of struggles with sinusitis, gastrointestinal disorders, and stress-related conditions, he embraced a journey of self-healing through lifestyle changes, balanced nutrition, and regular exercise. Inspired by the disciplined example of his late father and guided by holistic health principles, Rabi Narayan now enjoys an active and thriving life, free from illness.

With a professional background in Engineering and Business Administration, Rabi Narayan combines a scientific understanding of health with a practical approach to daily living. As a wellness coach, he helps individuals create sustainable habits that lead to holistic health transformations. Rabi Narayan also writes regularly on health and wellness topics, sharing research-backed insights through his own blog site and contributing to other respected platforms in the wellness community.

This book marks Rabi Narayan Mohanty's debut as an author, offering readers a roadmap to achieving optimal health through a blend of personal stories, practical advice, and proven wellness strategies. Whether you're looking to lose weight, eat better, or adopt healthier habits, this book provides a step-by-step guide to a more vibrant and balanced life.

DISCLAIMER

The information contained in this book is provided for educational and informational purposes only. It is not intended as medical advice, nor should it be used as a substitute for professional medical consultation, diagnosis, or treatment. Always seek the advice of your physician or other qualified health provider with any questions you may have regarding a medical condition or health concerns.

The author and publisher disclaim any liability for any adverse effects or consequences resulting from the use or application of any information or techniques described in this book. The content reflects the author's personal experiences and opinions and may not be applicable to everyone. Individual results may vary. The author makes no representations or warranties with respect to the accuracy or completeness of the contents of this work and specifically disclaims all warranties, including without limitation warranties of fitness for a particular purpose.

The book is intended to provide general information and guidance based on the author's research and experience. Readers are encouraged to make their own decisions and consult with appropriate professionals before making significant changes to their health or lifestyle.

May I Ask You For A Small Favor?

First, I want to thank you for reading this book. You could have chosen any other book, but you took mine, and I appreciate this. I hope you have at least a few actionable insights that will positively impact your daily life.

Can I ask for 30 seconds more of your time?

I'd love it if you could leave a review of the book. That will help me grow my readership by encouraging folks to take a chance on my books.

Keeping it straight - reviews are the lifeblood of any author. It will take less than a minute of your time but will tremendously help me reach out to more people.

If you liked this book, please consider posting an honest review on your preferred retailer. And I'd love to see your review. Thanks for your support.

Your Free Gift

Scan the QR code below to receive your FREE GIFT!

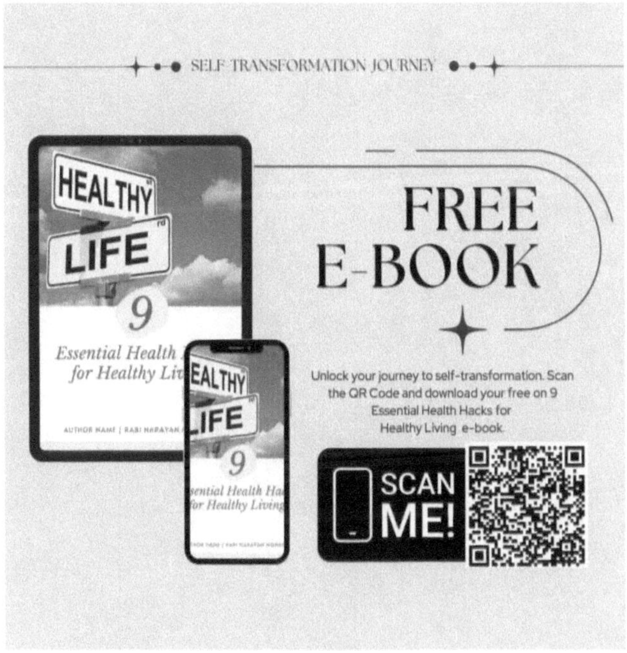